The Compass Method For Natural Weight Loss Without Complex Diets Or Strenuous Exercise

Dr. Chio Ugochukwu

**The Compass Method For Natural Weight Loss
Without Complex Diets Or Strenuous Exercise**

Published by Bundant Enterprises

3053 Rancho Blvd H-197
Palmdale, CA 93551

ISBN-13:978-1535078931

ISBN-10:1535078936

Printed in the United States of America

Disclaimer and Terms of Use

The author and publisher have made every effort to ensure the accuracy and completeness of information contained in this book, we assume no responsibility for errors or omissions therein. It is solely for informational and educational purposes and should not be regarded as a substitute for professional medical treatment, legal, tax or other professional advice. Your reliance upon information and content obtained through this book is solely at your own risk. The author and publisher assume no liability or responsibility for any adverse consequences for the use of any product, information, idea or instruction contained in the content provided to you through this book. Always consult your healthcare provider first.

Dedication

This book is dedicated to those who would like to learn easy and natural ways to lose weight and keep it off without relying on complex diets and strenuous exercises.

Acknowledgement

I would like to thank my lovely wife Ekene and my wonderful kids for their amazing support. I would also like to acknowledge the support and inspiration I get from those who read my books and share their thoughts and comments. We are all together in this journey of becoming better versions of ourselves. Finally, my gratitude goes to God, who makes all things beautiful in His time.

Table of Contents

Introduction

According to the CDC, more than 30% of people 19 years and older living in America are obese. Generally speaking, obese individuals are those who have a body mass index (BMI) of 30 or more. BMI is broadly divided into underweight(less than 18.5), normal weight (18.5 to 24.9), over weight (25.0 to 29.9), obesity (30.0 to 39.9) and morbid obesity (40.0 or higher). While morbid obesity is more associated with adverse health outcomes, obese and overweight individuals are still predisposed to health problems like colon cancer, coronary heart disease, diabetes and high blood pressure.

The reasons for losing weight can vary from health and medical reasons like diabetes, hypertension, arthritis, sleeping and breathing problems, to social reasons like becoming more active and having more fun or even personal ones like wanting to wear smaller size clothes. Apart from the well documented health reasons for losing weight, the process of losing weight and keeping it off, can help you become more energetic and confident. This will help you to be ready to regularly participate more enthusiastically in the activities of daily living.

Sadly, though most people are aware of the dangers or consequences of being overweight, including its association with health problems and reduced quality of life, few people are able to consistently implement those steps that will enable them lose weight and keep it off. Research has shown that 60-70% of people who begin to exercise, stop within 6-9 months (Ansel, 2010). Part of the reason why this happens is that most people with the intention to improve their health or lose weight try to make major changes to their lifestyle, without a better understanding of themselves, and their motivations.

Through this book, I will share with you, natural and easy ways, you can lose weight and keep it off, through a step by step process using the Compass Method, without relying on complex diets or strenuous exercise. **After reading this book you will be able to develop your own easy to implement Compass Hybrid Individualized Plan (CHIP) for weight loss.**

Learn more about how a deeper understanding of your personality, passion, strengths and weaknesses can help you lose weight

If you learn more about yourself, you will know more about your strengths and weaknesses and how they influence your decision making process. This will include learning more about your personality, passion, challenges and motivators. This will help you to become more confident in the actions you take. Without confidence in yourself, you will be prone to too many decision reversals and over reliance on other people's opinion.

Learning how to encourage yourself to succeed is an important part of the process of losing weight consistently or keeping it off. In order to do this you have to have to gain a better understanding of your strengths, weaknesses and fears. What are your deepest fears and worries? What is holding you back from taking action today? What is affecting your confidence in yourself and your ability to make decisions? What is holding you back from making a commitment to change yourself? Is it fear of the process or fear of failure? Don't forget that challenges and failures are part of your journey of success.

Asking or answering asking these questions will help you recognize your strengths, challenges and weaknesses. With a better understanding of yourself, you will be to stay focused on the process and take action even on the days everything seems to be working against you. **Do your best and leave the rest. The smallest action is better than the greatest intention.** Taking action will help you reduce stress and have more energy for all the fun things you would like to do with your life.

Nothing in life is perfect, so if you find some of these steps in the compass method for weight loss too hard to take, begin with the ones you find easier to do.

Learn how to analyze things for yourself, how to get things done and how you can continue to improve. The simplest way to do this is to look back at your life and find out which method of preparation and execution has worked the best for you in your most successful projects. You can then modify your weight-loss strategy to fit that model.

Part of learning more about yourself, would also include learning more about your personality. Your personality is generally accepted to mean the pattern of relatively permanent traits and unique characteristics that gives both consistency and individuality to the way you behave or function in different circumstances and situations (Feist & Feist, 2009). With this definition in mind, you can see why it will be important for you to make understanding your personality an important part of your individualized weight-loss plan.

According to Linda Malone, people with outgoing personalities like an "I" personality type or sanguine personality, tend to allow stress to accumulate to the point where their response to stress becomes dominated by pleasure-based eating. This is similar to trying to deal with stress by drinking alcohol. It does not work. Pleasure-based eating can lead one to eat too much pleasant tasting food like high-fat content food, and carbohydrate-rich foods like candy and cookies. These two options would lead to high calorie intakes that can lead to weight gain, unless you figure out how to reduce stress, before it triggers excessive eating.

The bottom line is you have to remember that your personality will influence your basic motivations for participating in different aspects of your daily life. This is why you have to take your personality type into consideration when crafting or implementing your own individualized natural weight-loss strategy through the Compass Method.

Knowing your passion is part of how you know yourself. This is because unless you have a better understanding of yourself, you will always stumble or have difficulty as you try to relate to others and to yourself.

Your passion is part of what connects you to the world. What one thing or item would you like to change in the world? Your answer here could be a multitude of things including providing better drinking water, helping underprivileged children, stopping cruelty to animals or making your neighborhood safer. The point is that if you do not stay healthy by losing weight, you will not be able to follow your passion. This is why you have to make getting motivated by your passion the cornerstone of your individualized pan to lose weight.

You can also discover you passion by asking yourself relevant questions about what you like to do in your spare time. You probably spend time doing things you are passionate about. You may spend time hiking, writing, playing music, exercising or doing whatever you enjoy. If you really want to lose weight easily and keep it off, you have to make your weight-loss strategies and activities part of what you like.

What makes you smile? All those things that make you smile are things that you love and enjoy doing. Of course, it doesn't have to be an item. Spending time with your grandchildren or visiting a senior home can be other things that put a smile on your face.

Go through this list and start writing down your answers. From here you want to see if there is one thing that gets repeated again and again. If so, chances are that this is your passion.

By finding your passion and making it a greater part of your life, you will enjoy more of your daily activities and cut down on stress. This will help you reduce the tendency to eat snacks to cope with daily emotional pains. I know I have had to frequently deal with this problem myself until I finally came to accept my passion and the challenges that are associated with it. Do not expect everyone close to you to show love and understanding towards you because you have discovered your passion, motivation or the benefits of daily exercise. Why are you doing what you are doing?

Focus more on your strengths and take daily action to help you lose weight so that can feel good about yourself and enjoy your hobbies and interests. **Take action that will help your talents and gifts flourish instead of worrying about your weaknesses and what other people have to say about you.**

The more you use your passion to focus on the positive, the less stressed out you will be. The less stressed out you are, the less you will be tempted to use eating as a way to cope with your emotional challenges. The more you can manage or control what you eat the more you can lose weight in a sustainable way. Next you need to learn about how to use the compass profiles to gain a deeper understanding of yourself and facilitate your weight-loss strategy.

Action Tips

Find out more about how personality type contributes to your daily choices and decisions

If you want to learn more about your

DISC personality visit;

http://www.compasswellnessinstitute.com/your-disc-personality-profile/

Ask questions that will help you discover your passion and motivation

Make your passion the anchor reason why you want to lose weight

Find out your personality type

Use the compass profiles to understand yourself better and facilitate your weight loss

The compass health profiles are the foundation for the Compass Method for transformational living. You can apply the method to your natural weight-loss strategy. The first component of the compass profile is **community relationships.**

The first step in relating to others is relating to yourself. If you do not take good care of yourself, you may find yourself too cranky and lethargic to take care of others. Communicate with yourself first and write down your deepest fears and worries. What is holding you back from being the best version of yourself? What is affecting your confidence in yourself and your ability to make decisions? Are you always looking for approval and validation from others? What is holding you back from making a commitment to change yourself? Is it fear of failure, or fear of the process and communication?

Good communication is good because it helps to reduce stress. If you feel you are not good at it, don't let it bother you. **Don't let the perfect become the enemy of the possible.** Taking action will help you reduce stress and have more energy for all the fun things you would like to do with your life. Nothing in life is perfect, so if you find some of these steps too hard to take, begin with the actions you can take today.

Answering or asking these questions will help you recognize which aspects of your relationship with others could either be contributing to your weight gain or making it more difficult for you to lose weight. Just remember that you can also make your friends part of your family. After all, good companionship from those we live with and interact with everyday helps us live longer and better.

This requires a lot of give and take. Through your **operational capacity profile,** you will learn how to analyze things for yourself, how to get things done and how you can continue to improve. The simplest way to do this is to look back at your life and find out which method of preparation and execution has worked the best for you in your most successful projects. You can then modify your weight-loss strategy to fit that model.

If one of your weaknesses is getting things done in the last minute, then it means you tend to procrastinate and underestimate how much time you would need to get things done. Remember that inadequate preparation leads to failure. To lose weight and keep it off, you will have to start with a small plan and build on it slowly, in a way that takes advantage of your strengths while minimizing your weaknesses.

You can get your **metabolic analysis** by getting your physiological and laboratory tests done. This will help you to know if there are significant medical problems responsible for your weight. Getting the right tests done with the help of a healthcare professional or your doctor will make it easy for you to know which aspect of your health profile you need to focus on improving.

When it comes to losing weight even without running tests, **your family history can help you a get a better** picture of your risk factors. Studies have shown that being overweight and obese run in families (National Heart, Lung and blood Institute).If you have a family history of diabetes or chronic obesity then you have to be much more vigilant than others. This is because most of these disease conditions run in families and make the process of losing weight more challenging.

The Physical Profile includes your weight, height, waist circumference and BMI (Body Mass Index). It also includes your heart rate and lung function. These factors are important because it is important to know your health status before you can engage in vigorous exercise. **Take action today, weigh yourself today, even if you feel you are in excellent health.**

The main exercise protocol proposed in **the Compass Method** is mild to moderate activities like **walking**, dancing, jump ropes and pushups. If you are more used to vigorous activities like playing basketball, tennis, and baseball, you need to remember to check with your doctor to make sure that you are healthy enough to continue to exercise vigorously. One advantage of staying physically active is that it helps you burn off excessive energy that would have been converted to fat. Increased storage of excess energy in the form of fat will ultimately build up your weight and cause more health problems.

The Ambition profile looks at how you try to improve yourself, your job and finances and satisfaction with your life. This is important because without good finances or insurance it is much more difficult to take good care of your health. The ambition profile measures your ability to get things done or to make adjustments when they are required. **Set measurable goals like reducing your weight by 10Lbs with a projected time-frame to help you implement the process. This is an important bench mark because once you can confidently write down the actions and activities that helped you lose your first 10 pounds, you can build on it to lose more pounds.**

The remaining two profiles are **Spirituality and Self Knowledge**, both of which examine your psychospiritual make up. They will help you have a **better understanding of your personality,** character and connection with God and the universe, depending on what you believe. The bottom line is that **knowing more about your personality type will give you a greater insight into how your personality affects your weight loss strategy.** Though there are many classifications or names for different personality types, **the DISC personality profile is the one used in the Compass Method.**

A better understanding of your strengths and weaknesses will help you know your limitations, when it comes to deciding on the easy ways consistent self-improvement and thriving more. It will also help you to anticipate problems, quarrels and pressure points.

On the spiritual side of the equation, more and more studies are beginning to show that those who meditate or are truly prayerful are better able to handle health challenges than those who do neither. Of course I realize that there are different interpretations of what it means to be spiritual and that one size does not fit all. Next we shall begin the whole process by adjusting your eating habits so that you can lose weight through sustainable lifestyle changes.

Action Tips

Write down a paragraph that best explains your best understanding of yourself, including your strengths and weaknesses

Adjust your eating habits so that you can lose weight through sustainable lifestyle changes

The problem most people have is that they get so caught up with trying new ways of eating healthy that they give up before they get the results they want. This can be very discouraging and frustrating. The whole process may even feel like torture.

Instead of torturing yourself by chasing the latest complicated diet fad, adjust what you eat everyday to what is healthy and enjoyable to you. This is part of the Compass Method and it is based on the idea that it will be easier to make adjustments to the food you are used to eating than to try to acquire a new taste. Most people that begin a new diet find it hard to sustain and end up quitting before they can lose weight.

The first step to take in adjusting your eating habits would be to cut down the servings or portions of your regular meal by half. This will reduce your energy intake by about half or a third. You fill the gap with vegetables and fruits. **If you feel pangs of hunger, snack with nuts, drink plenty of water or eat some fruits.**

The more your servings are reduced, the more weight you would lose because the fewer calories you will take in, the more energy will be obtained from excess body fat resulting in weight loss. However, reduced servings may mean more hunger pangs. This is a serious potential problem that sometimes makes people drink a lot of soda or eat many hot dogs as an immediate way of dealing with their hunger pangs. This simply leads to more energy intake and more weight gain.

To deal with this, eat more fruits, vegetables and fibers as fillers. Fibers are especially good for your system because they help to increase bowel movement. This has the added effect of making your digestive system more efficient.

For different cultures and settings, different modifications to familiar eating habits can be made. In America this would entail cutting down on fast foods, soda and other processed foods. You can do this by going to eat fast food only once a month. If you cannot do this, start by either eating only small sizes or eating only half of the sandwich that you buy.

Do not go along with food choices that will not be good for your health just because people from your culture may challenge you or make fun of you. Your culture is supposed to help you, not to kill you. You can do this by finding a way to eat right within your culture.

Do a 72-hour food audit before you make the final decision on your adjustments. You can do this by simply writing down the food, drinks and snacks you have eaten in the past 72 hours. Through your food audit, you will know what food dominates your eating pattern and what adjustments you need to make. When I did my food audit, I found out that my eating pattern was dominated by rice and bread. I made changes. I added more, corn, fruits and nuts to my daily food.

I also found out through my food audit that while my goal was to reduce sodium intake to about 1500 mg per day and cut down my energy intake by half. The challenge to this goal was that while I was able to quickly reduce my food portions, I found myself snacking too much everyday. I was eating about 10 slices of bread everyday. This meant I was already getting too much sodium and calories just from bread alone without even adding my other sources of sodium. On the average a slide of bread contains 150 mg of sodium and 110 calories per serving. This would mean that for bread with one slice per serving, 10 slices would be 1100 calories. This would be more than the average 2000 calories per day recommended for most people.

Finally, I figured out why despite my reduction in portions, regular exercise and eating fruits and vegetables my weight loss was slow and inconsistent. To make matters worse, I had been using nuts for snacks without checking their sugar content and calories per serving. One small pack of unsalted pea nuts contained 220 calories per serving but 6 servings per pack. Don't worry, you do not have to count calories to learn this! You simply have to form the habit of consistently reading your nutrition facts.

This shows that though I had reduced my calories per meal through reducing my portion per meal, because I had not paid careful attention to size or frequency of my snacks, I was eating a lot of calories per day through snacks. As soon as I discovered this, I cut my snack portions by half and cut down my slices of bread to, not more than 4 per day. This helped me reduce my extra calories by more than half. This adjustment helped me to start losing weight more consistently and keeping it off. **If you want to lose weight, you have to know your daily sources of extra calories and eliminate them.**

All you have to do is to remember that you have to reduce all sources of your daily intake of calories from your meals to your snacks. Do this to a level that allows you to feel full, eat healthy and still lose weight.

According to Dr. Wang an energy intake and expenditure expert, consistent loss or reduction in energy intake of 100 calories would lead to 10 pounds loss in weight (Reuters Health, 2015). **This means that without knowing the exact quantity of calories you eat, you can continue to reduce your meal, snack or social eating portions until you notice your first loss of 10 pounds and use it for a marker or foundation for all your future weight-loss strategies.**

Research has shown that drinking water before a meal will help to expand your stomach. This approach will make you feel completely full when you are only 80% full. This is important because eating only up to 80 % full was one of the common practices of people of Okinawa in Japan, who have the highest number of centenarians in the world. My suggestion is that you drink at least two glasses of water per meal and increase the bulk in your meals through fruits and vegetables. **This will help you reduce your total calorie intake per meal without tortures diets.** You can do this by increasing your daily intake of salads consisting of cabbage, tomatoes, carrots, broccoli, spinach and bananas. Eating a colorful variety of fruits and vegetables per meal with reduced portions of your regular main meal will significantly more your food more healthy and more bulky but less energy dense. This will help you to significant lose pounds and keep them off. **Remember calories in calories out.**

You need to be careful when you start cutting down on calories by reducing the intake of carbohydrate like white bread, white rice or pasta. This will make you lose weight quickly because it is usually stored in the body as glycogen which contains water. You need to be careful because the brain gets most of its energy from glucose and if it does not get enough you begin to feel tired, weak, unable to sleep and ill. Unless you switch to fiber-rich carbohydrate sources like baked sweet potato, whole grain bread, barley, oat meal and brown rice, you may end up quitting after a few weeks. This is why **the compass method is focused on adjustments and individualized modifications**.

Whatever you decide, start small. Remember that little drops of water make the mighty ocean. This thought will help you, even when you feel overwhelmed by the thought of changing your eating habits. When I changed my eating habits, I started by making small changes like adding salads to every meal of rice that I had. I found the whole idea difficult initially but I had to remind myself the passion behind my decision to lose weight. Try a few combinations to find out what will work best for you.

To make sustainable adjustments and modifications to your meals concentrate on making aggregate changes. Include chicken, fish, beans, cottage cheese, or low fat yogurt in your meals. Have eggs, nuts and red meat occasionally. You can further reduce your fat intake by eating skinless chicken or turkey. Turkey and chicken have their fat on their skin but red meat has most of its fat contained within the meat. Grilling is better than frying, and always aim to use unsaturated oils like corn, and olive oils for cooking.

You can also gradually reduce the fat content in your milk products. You can do this by changing from whole milk, to 2% fat; then to 1% fat. Fat free milk is not recommended because it is still important to get fat in your body which can be used through cellular metabolism to produce cell membranes and hormones. Choose lower-fat cheese and yogurt. When you buy yogurt, also check that it does not contain sugar. The good thing about reducing to 1% fat milk is that it remains tasteful. Fat has 9 calories of energy per gram compared to carbohydrate and proteins that have about 4 per gram.

Mix up your selection of meals so that you can look forward to your meal time. Do not eat the same meal day in day out. Why? It gets boring after a while and you will soon find yourself looking less forward to eating healthy.

Make sure your food contains adequate but moderate portions of fat, proteins, carbohydrates and vitamins. Eat enough food to fill full, when you eat. If you don't feel full after a meal you will find yourself eating too much sugary snacks in between meals to make you feel full. This will make you gain back weight you may have lost. If you feel hungry between meals, snack with small portions of almonds, cashew nuts or peanuts. Almonds will make you feel less hungry and still boost your metabolism.

Eat everything in moderation. Do not eat a particular food too much just because you like it. Concentrate on eating non-processed food instead of on processed food like bacon and "ready-to-go" meals like frozen burritos and pizzas. They are convenient but have high sugar and high dense calories! These will make you gain weight fast. Remember that our goal is to eat as much food as we can in their natural state.

Be particularly careful with how much soda or beer you drink. Beer has a lot of calories with little ingredients. Drinking too much beer may cost you some important vitamins like vitamin B 6. Another way to balance your meal would be to halve your intake of all pure or added fats as previously outlined.

Plan your meals and snacks ahead of time. Take time to plan at least one lunch and dinner every week without meat or cheese. Build those meals around whole grains, vegetables and beans to increase fiber and reduce fat. If you want to have something to chew on, get some nuts, fish or tofu. You can make every Friday your fish meal day. If you have a plan, stick to it. Learn to say, "No" at social gatherings when friends and company will try to tease you to eat food you already know from experience will not work for you.

Have at least five servings of fruit every day. This can be for dessert or snacks. Choose fruit that is in season. My rule is to take an apple per meal. If you can, go for those red delicious apples because they contain pectin, a fiber that helps to promote healthy cholesterol levels and contain more amounts of antioxidants than many other types of apples.

Apart from the adjustments that affect food portion and type of food eaten, the other adjustment you can make to your eating habits would include eating slowly and eating without watching TV. One way you can get yourself to eat more slowly and enjoy your food more is to find a place where you eat on a regular basis everyday. This could be eating breakfast at home, instead of in your car. If due to your busy schedule you cannot do this in the morning then make it a priority at other meal times. The key is that you have to focus on doing one thing at a time. **Instead of sitting in front of the TV after work , eating and watching TV, sit at your dining table and eat your super slowly. Next read your nutrition facts.**

Action Tips

Do your 72-hour food audit

Cut down your serving portions for meals

Eat food that is rich in fruits and whole grains

Modify your typical cultural food

Drink two glasses of water before every meal

Eat an apple per meal

Plan your snacks in advance

Cut down on your snack portions

Cut down on soda and beer

Eat slowly

Do not eat and watch TV at the same time

Avoid processed food as much as you can

Eat natural

Make reading your nutritional facts part of your strategy for natural weight loss

Though the emphasis of the Compass Method for adjusting your diet is on eating food as natural as possible, we recognize that there are certain times when we all have to eat food that has been processed in one form or another. This will include breakfast cereals, fruit juices or even some pre-packaged meals. The key is to read your nutrition facts whenever you have to eat food that comes in a box, container or package.

You have to look at reading your nutritional facts the same way you look at reading or looking at your gas or fuel gauge in your car. If you do not form the habit of checking your gas gauge in your car, you could end up with an empty tank in the middle of nowhere or in a very dangerous part of town. If you do not read your nutrition facts you may end up unwittingly eating food that could make you gain weight or worse still turn out to be very dangerous to your health.

Reading your nutritional facts will give you an idea of the quantity, food types and ingredients in the food you eat everyday. This will help you know how much calories, carbohydrate, fat, protein and sodium is in the food you eat. Physiologically sodium which is the main component of salt draws in water wherever it is found in the body. This means that if you do not watch your total sodium intake, you may unwittingly expose yourself to daily fluctuations in your weight, depending on how much water you retain.

This usually happens because other sources of sodium have not been accounted for. This includes salt used in cooking and salt used in preserving pre-cooked food. The first is obvious while the second will involve some research. Unfortunately, most of us do not have time for research so we just end up eating with sounds healthy and move on.

The problem is that without taking the time to read our nutritional labels we could end up eating more fluid-retaining-food or food high in calories without knowing it. Do you know how much salt is contained in pre-cooked burrito? On average one burrito has 470mg to 1200mg of sodium. These are significant numbers especially, if you are trying to keep your daily sodium intake to 1500mg of sodium or less. If you do not watch your sodium intake by taking time to read your nutrition facts, you could end up eating much more sodium than you planned.

Generally, when I look at my nutrition facts, I look at my sodium, potassium, fiber, sugar, calories and fat content. I know people sometimes ignore their sodium content, thinking it does not really matter. Well, it does. When comparing a loaf of bread with a can of soda, you will find that on average a single serving of bread contains 150 milligrams of sodium, while the can of soda contains 65 milligrams of sodium per serving size.

The other important facts you will learn about the food you are about to eat by looking at the food label, would be how much sugar it has, and the calories per serving. This is important because you need to cut down you calorie intake to lose weight. Studies have shown that it is easier to lose weight by reducing energy intake, than by trying to use exercise and physical activity to burn off excess energy intake after eating too much. **Unless you** get this principle clear and apply it daily to your weight loss strategies, you will fail. This is the principle of calories in, calories out.

If you enjoy eating bread because of its fibers you may unwittingly be eating too much sodium or eating sugar. A serving of bread, which is usually one or two slices, also contains on average 3g of sugar. According to the American Heart Association (AHA), the recommended sugar intake for men is 37.5g and for women 25g. This means that if you eat 8 servings of bread, you would have eaten 24g of sugar. The increase in sugar in your body can lead to an increase in your triglycerides and lead to a reduction in the level of high density lipoproteins (HDL) in your body.

By reading your food facts you will know how much sodium or sugar each choice you make will add to your daily energy intake. All you need is a broad idea, you do not need to count calories or know the percentage daily value of everything you eat. This type of knowledge will ultimately help you to control or reduce your total calories without putting too much effort into it.

The more you know about the daily factors that can affect your weight, and take action, the more you will be able to eat healthy in a smart way that works for you, without getting on torture diets. Next you have to make increased physical activity part of your daily strategy for losing weight and keep it off.

Action Tips

Start reading your nutrition facts
Cut down on your total sodium intake and not just added salt
Cut down on your daily sugar intake

Make increased physical activity part of your daily strategy for losing weight and keeping it off

You need to make a conscious effort to increase your daily physical activity. This would include deliberately looking for ways to participate in physical activities at home, at work and in social gatherings. At home make out time garden or to mow the lawn yourself instead of giving out as a contract to others. You could also participate more in yard cleaning, every little bit counts. At social gatherings, volunteer to clean up and move the chairs and tables. At work or at events, walk up and down the stairs instead of using the elevators or lift. Remember that little drops of water make the mighty ocean.

Increased daily physical activity has the metabolic effect of helping you burn off energy everyday, so that there is less excess energy left in the body to be converted to fat for storage. This means you will gain less weight.

You can also increase physical activity by doing something as simple as walking to as many places as you can everyday. First, make sure it is safe. As you go through your daily activities, make it a point to walk a little further. One of my favorite tricks for doing this is to park far away from the entrance each time I go to the grocery store or the mall. This will help you take a few more steps everyday. Try it. You will be surprised at how effective this can become for you without changing your lifestyle a great deal.

There are several different exercises or physical activities that you can do to help you burn off more energy and minimize the effects of daily stress in your life. Walking is among the best, as you can easily lose yourself and your troubles by walking. Even if it is just around the block, walking can do wonders for your health. It can also help to reduce your stress level.

If you have a lot of stress in your life, you may want to consider a gym or doing yoga stretches at home. Working out and then sitting in the sauna is also a good way to relieve tension. It will also help you sweat a lot and lose more weight. First you have to make sure you are healthy enough by asking your doctor if you can use a sauna.

If you do not like walking or going to the gym, consider going for swimming exercises, joining a dance class or even playing tennis. If you have a pool at home, you may find swimming to be very beneficial way to increase physical activity and help you relax. Focus on low impact exercises and avoid strenuous exercises that can easily damage your body.

If you find yourself doing a lot of standing or sitting as part of your job or daily life, then find ways to break the monotony every 2 hours. Do this even if it means simply getting up and walking around in your office or simply stretching from time to time. It may also be as simple as rolling your seat back and bending down to pick up a pen or piece of paper, without using a pick up stick or asking for help.

The bottom line is that if you find any exercise pattern that fits into your life style and do it regularly, you will see that the pounds will start falling off gradually. Increased daily physical activity will help you increase your level of daily metabolism without making any special effort. On the other hand, if you spend most of your days, sitting in the car, sitting down at work in the office, and sitting down in front of the TV or internet at home, then your daily metabolism will be low and you will   find yourself gradually gaining more weight.

I am not saying become a weekend warrior and try to build a tree house every weekend. The key emphasis is on simplistic and sustainability. Start with increasing your daily physical activity like mowing your lawn, cleaning your house, washing your car and going for daily walks. Aim for a combined total of about 45 minutes of physical activity most days of the week. Next do not overlook the importance of doing consistent daily exercise in helping you lose weight and keep it off.

Action Tips

Make increased physical activity part of your daily lifestyle

Write down three more things you could do differently in your daily routine that will help you to become physically more active

Learn to use consistent daily low impact exercise to help you lose weight naturally

I will share with you how becoming more consistent in my daily exercise routine helped me with my weight-loss strategy. The goal was to lose 10 pounds in six weeks. I started by walking briskly for at least 45 minutes, at least five times a week. I started by walking 30 minutes a day for the first week, then I increased it to 45 minutes a day.

After about 2 weeks, I found it difficult to consistently create the 45 minutes block of time, so I changed to 3 blocks of 15 minute-time intervals everyday. The advantage of this approach was that I found it easier to create 15 minute-time blocks for daily exercise. If your target is 60 minutes of exercise everyday, you can break it up into 20 minutes each. I gradually incorporated these changes into my daily routine and into my lifestyle. This helped me become more energetic and more confident. More importantly it helped me trust the process. Trusting the process, and making daily adjustments helped me become more consistent in the reaming 4 weeks of my 6-week weight loss challenge and I ended up making my goal of losing 10 pounds in six weeks.

If you plan to use walking as the main part of your daily exercise be prepared to make adjustments. As you get older you will begin to notice a tiny but perceptible bulge in your waist line that is usually due to reduced metabolism and reduced muscle mass. It is belly fat and if you do not pay attention to it, it will continue to grow and add to your weight.

If you are struggling with belly fat, you have to include exercises that will further strengthen your muscles, to your daily exercise routine. This is important because after 40 years of age, muscle strength becomes weaker. If you fail to take action to strengthen your muscles, you will end up with a more protruding belly and gradually gaining back the weight you had lost initially after you started walking. You can do this by participating in muscle strengthening activities like playing leisure tennis, ping pong, walking with extra weights, jogging, doing pushups and jump ropes every week. Choose one of these or any other similar one that will work best for your personality, experience and schedule. The key thing is to choose a low impact exercise that is not too strenuous for you and do it consistently.

Remember that for men the waist circumference measured above the hip bones while relaxed and exhaling should not be more than 40 inches or 100cm and for women not more than 35 inches or 88cm.The exception is pregnancy for women.

One of the reasons we gain belly fat as we get older is that we worry about more things than we did as teenagers or young adults. You now have to worry about your job, your mortgage, your children's education and your in-laws. New sources of stress mean more release of cortisol, the stress hormone. Cortisol leads to the distribution of fat into the abdominal area, making a bad situation worse. Cortisol will also cause the retention of sodium and will lead to increase in water retention and your weight.

One of the simplest and natural ways you can lose weight through low impact exercise is do push ups everyday. You can do this by doing at least 50 pushups every day. Instead of trying to do 50 at a time, start by doing 10 pushups at a time. After each ten, take a 1 to 3 minute break, then continue until you have completed 50 pushups. If you cannot do it all in one session break it up into two or three sessions that you find comfortable. If 50 a day is too high a target for you, start with 20 a day. Do not exceed 50 a day and do you pushups on alternate days, to give your muscles time to recover and grow.

These muscle-strengthening exercises will help you increase your muscle mass as well as increase your total energy expenditure and reduce the amount of excess energy to be converted to visceral or stomach fat. No matter which muscle strengthening exercise you decide to use, take time to warm up before you begin to exercise and cool down after exercise. This will help to protect your heart. It is always a good idea to first discuss your exercise plans with your doctor or healthcare professional before you begin. Take time to draw your own weight loss pie chart. It will help you monitor your progress. Next use concurrent adjustments to manage daily stress and keep your focus on losing weight.

Action tips

Do your daily exercise

Focus on the process

Measure your waist circumference

Weigh yourself everyweek

Use concurrent adjustments to manage daily stress and maintain your focus on losing weight

There are factors and activities throughout the day that can affect our emotional well-being. These include time management, Negative conversations, money-issues, relationship conflicts, anxiety and anger. These are potentially sources of daily stress that can our minds off our best intentions and lead us away from an effective weight-loss strategy. The truth is that we all have problems or things we do not do well and our emotions play a big role on how we respond to our daily circumstances.

One of the best ways we can protect our emotional well-being and manage daily stress is to expect the unexpected. Each one of us must find ways to deal with those times when people return kindness with rudeness, fairness with unfairness. Whenever I encounter such situations, I remind myself that how I react is more important than whatever is said by someone else. I begin my "gratitude" mantra to help me relax and reduce emotional tension. I purposely become grateful for obvious daily activities like eating, walking, smiling, talking and being able to read small print.

We have to learn how to deal with our social and physical environment. We also have to learn how to interact with others and how we deal with our deepest fears. If we don't get it right, we build up stress that will ultimately affect our sleep, heart and digestive systems. This can lead to sleepless nights and overeating.

We can empower ourselves to deal with such circumstances by reminding yourself that people lash out or say mean things when they feel frustrated, insecure, uncomfortable or unappreciated. This is just an emotional outburst. Do not take such outbursts personal. If you take them personal they will affect your ability to stay focused on your weight-loss strategy and achieve your desired daily objectives in terms of process.

Instead treat each outburst or episode as an opportunity to be thankful. Anticipate 5 daily humiliations, setbacks or toxic emotional outbursts from your interactions with others everyday. Have a strategy for dealing with them before they arise. You can decide to count their occurrences everyday.

One of the ways to empower yourself is to learn your emotional triggers and have strategies to deal with such situations before they arise or as soon as they arise. Self-knowledge, which is one of the seven dimensions of the compass health profile, will definitely enable us to empower ourselves and live more healthy lives. Knowing your DISC personality will help. The ways we can do this varies broadly because of our different personalities, circumstances, and spiritual outlooks. We have to recognize that despite our best efforts to focus on losing weight without complexities, stress and conflicts will always be are part our relationships at home, work or social gatherings.

How we feel affects how we see ourselves and how we interact with others. If we do not feel good about ourselves, we are less likely to do those things that will help us lose weight and make us truly happy. For example, being in a bad mood can make us decide to skip the fruits and salads that we know will help us lose weight and stay healthy. Worse still, you may feel so bad that you end up drinking and smoking. These types of negative behaviors will make it more difficult for you to lose weight unless you manage our daily stress better.

According to a study from the University of Alabama, those who ate in response to an emotional stress were 13 times more likely to be overweight or obese. We all know the additional health risks associated with being overweight.

Another source of daily stress is imbalance between our relationships and finances. The right balance between your finances, relationships and health will help you to reduce stress and accomplish your daily weight-loss objectives and goals. When you set your weight loss goals you have to pursue its fulfillment through consistent daily action. Do not let unexpected the twists and turns of daily life keep you from taking consistent action in the different spheres that constitute your daily life.

If we fail to strike the right balance between our work and our relationships then there will be a buildup of stress and illness in our lives. We shall find ourselves quick to anger and less tolerant of others and their mistakes. **We shall find ourselves less able to concentrate and maintain the discipline that will help us to watch what we eat, exercise when we should or let go of daily irritations.**

How much balance do you have in your life? To find out how much balance you have in your life spend fifteen minutes of your day, examining how much time you spend on your finances, relationships, and health. How much time do you put into making your weight-loss strategy a priority in your daily life without making other aspects of your life suffer? If you do not strike the right balance and build harmony in your life and environment through your weight-loss strategy, your success will be limited and unsustainable.

Action tips

Say 10 positive thoughts everyday

Lower your expectations from others

Forgive and forgive and again

What is your balance time bar chart?

What aspect of your life costs you the most time everyday?

Cut down on expenses for participating fully in preventive care

Avoid making the mistake of taking conversational stress for granted when you are trying to lose weight

Your daily conversations are an important part of your daily life. It is through them that you relate to friends, family and co-workers. It can also be a source of stress and anxiety.

Coping with conversational stress is important because we interact with others through our conversations with them. We do this by listening to others, talking to others and responding to what others say or have failed to say or do. Unless we are able to make the distinction between what needs a response what does not, we may end up getting worked up.

A simple strategy for coping with the potential emotional tension that may sometimes arise from our daily conversations would be to divide our conversations or activities into "little rocks" and "heavy rocks". Little rocks are those conversations you can either overlook or can decide to ignore without losing out significantly. What is an example of little rock conversation? If you are in the midst of a conversation with your brother and he is arguing that the sun goes round the earth, what will you say? Will you continue to argue even when you have shown him irrevocable evidence and he continues to argue? Arguing for arguing sake will only get you worked up and build up your stress level. This is an example of the "Little rocks" in a conversation. Let it go! **You don't have to have the last word.**

If you do not let it go, stress will build up and lead to the release of hormones that will make you store more fat. Corticosteroids which are released by the adrenal gland during stress can lead to increase in belly fat and weight gain.

You have more important things to do with your time and energy than getting into conversations that do not enhance your sense of well-being. **Instead learn to focus on your main goals in each conversational encounter. Ignore those who like to put you down on get into quarrels and point making.**

Create time to take care of your daily "big rocks". Spending quality time with your family should be considered a 'big rock". You could go and watch a movie with your friend, wife or partner. You could go swimming or go for a walk in the park. You could spend more time working on projects or goals that mean a lot to you. Next make an effort to sleep more adequately everyday.

Action Tips

Sometimes you win by loosing

Make an effort to sleep more adequately everyday

Sometimes we are so caught up in our work, entertainment and daily activities that we put adequate daily sleep on the back burner. The problem is that if do not sleep well everyday, our internal balance gets misaligned and the different organ systems in our body begin to function out of step. This will ultimately lead to more stress and less efficient metabolism that will make you gain weight or sabotage your efforts at losing weight.

On the other hand, sleeping more adequately will help you lose weight and keep it off. As we get older we discover that sleep does not come as readily as in the past. The other problem is that with more responsibilities and more obligations more people sacrifice or postpone adequate sleep for increased daily activity. The problem is that inadequate sleep will eventually affect your health and productivity.

One way most people try to deal with insomnia is to take sleeping pills. The other way is start drinking too much coffee everyday. Neither of these approaches works at the core problem of inadequate sleep.

A better approach would be to make an effort to increase daily sleep through better time management and increased daily exercise. If you want to have more adequate sleep increase the amount of physical exercise that you participate in during the day. This is one of the key ways to help you get a good sleep at night. The more active your body is during the day, the more likely you are to relax at night and fall asleep faster.

If you doubt this, watch your children. You will find out they sleep the most, when they have been most busy running around and actively playing all day. They get into bed and fall sound asleep.

With regular exercise you'll notice that your quality of sleep is improved and the transition between the cycles and phases of sleep will become smoother and more regular. By keeping up your physical activity during the day, you may find it easier to deal with the stress and worries of your life.

Research and studies indicate that there is a direct correlation between how much we exercise and how we feel afterwards. You should try and increase your physical activity during the day. The goal here is to give your body enough stimulation during the day so that you aren't full of energy at night.

Your body requires a certain amount of physical activity in order to keep functioning in a healthy manner. It is also important to note that you should not be exercising one or two hours before you go to bed. Make your own individualized time-frame based on your experience.

The ideal exercise time is in the late afternoon or early evening. You want to make sure you expend your physical energy long before it is time for your body to rest and ready itself for sleep.

Apart from exercise, the other factors that contribute to poor sleep include watching too much TV and using your mobile devices late at night. This is part of the problem with poor time management. Don't stay up late to watch your favorite show. You may enjoy your show but you will end up not sleeping well at night. This will not be good for your weight especially if you are over 40 years old.

According to Cleland, Schmidt, Dwyer, &Venn, (2008) time spent in behaviors that involve a lot of sitting with little activity, like watching or viewing TV was thought to be one of the factors responsible for increasing number of people that are either overweight or obese in different parts of the world. The study also found that in both men and women the average time spent watching television increased with the increasing frequency of consuming food and drinks while watching television. Soft drink consumption during television viewing was associated with a greater increase in abdominal obesity in both men and women.

Apart from the weight gained from inactivity, eating and watching TV at the same time will make you have a less restful sleep. Next learn to use easy-to-implement strategies to make your weight-loss plan flexible.

Action Tips

Write down a rough estimate of how many minutes you exercise every week

Turn off your devices before you go to bed

Make a note of when you get to bed at night and when you wake up

Aim to sleep cumulatively 8 hours every day

Visit membership at www.compasswellnessinstitute.com to learn even more ways to help you sleep more adequately everyday

Use easy-to-implement strategies to keep your weight-loss plan flexible

First, be realistic do not try to lose 100 pounds in two days or one week. This is very hard to do in an enjoyable and practical manner. Losing weight is not the same as starvation. A more realistic goal might be losing 10 pounds in one month or 6 weeks.

If you want to lose weight in a manner that will last, you have to have strategies that will help make your weight-loss related activities fun to do. If not you will start then stop. Sometimes, I have to chuckle at how we concentrate too much on the total amount of pounds we have to lose, instead of finding simple and easy ways to lose a few pounds per week. In order to lose weight and keep it off, you have to do it in a way that is fun for you, easy to do and can be made part of your long-term healthy lifestyle.

Once you discover what works for you that you can do consistently, your weight loss will occur naturally. **By following the approaches discussed so far in this book you will discover your own individualized plan that is easy for you to implement**.

Second, remember the reason why you want to lose weight. Remind yourself of this reason regularly. This has to be the central passion that drives the activities you participate in, everyday to help you lose weight. You already know that you do not want to spend your old age in nursing homes suffering from one chronic illness after another. You want to have fun and age gracefully.

Third, do not worry about results. Concentrate on actually doing or taking the steps you set up in your simple plan for losing weight. If your plan requires walking 60 minutes a day, do it. Do not make excuses. If you are too busy to spare chunks of 60 minutes at a time, then cut it down to 20 minutes at a time.

Fourth, do not think like a child. Do not think that it is either you are getting everything right or everything is wrong. If you plan to walk 60 minutes a day but due to circumstances beyond your control you were able to do only 25 minutes, you have not failed. Do the 25 minutes that day, then do 95 minutes the next day. This still makes a total of 120 minutes in two days. On the third day you can go back to 60 minutes a day. Be flexible.

Fifth, make sure you keep track of your progress. Weigh yourself before you start then weigh yourself after every week. You can use a simple scale to weigh yourself. Measuring your weight regularly is one of the easiest checks on how your individualized health plan is working. It is easier to do than calculating your BMI or measuring your waist circumference. Just climb on a scale and read your weight.

If on the other hand you discover that you have gained back some of the weight you had lost, then do a quick 72 –hour food audit to see the eating patterns that are making you gain weight. Short-term weight gains usually are as a result of increasing calorie intake or eating more food, rather than simply from reducing physical activity.

The last time I discovered I was gaining back some weight through such a review, I discovered that I had a problem with snacks. I eat too much bread at night when I did not feel like sleeping though I needed to be sleeping. This was a bad idea and I only found out early because I had formed the habit of weighing myself every week. I was able to catch my weight gain and go back to my own individualized plan for weight loss. I replaced the late night snacks with small portions of nuts and banana.

A lapse is not a relapse. A mistake is not a failure. If you find yourself not sticking to your fruits and vegetables, think about trying out new fruits that you have not tried in the past. Talk to your support group, and share your ideas on eating time and food variety. Try again if you do not succeed the first time. If you are living by yourself and are longer in touch with your family or old friends, create a new support group or join one online.

Finally, do not forget to talk to your doctor or health care provider about your medications. Make sure you are not taking any medications that may make you gain weight. This is particularly important if through a chart of your weekly weight measurement you discover you have either been gaining weight or not losing weight as much as you expected.

Losing weight and maintaining your weight within the normal range for your age and height is certainly one of the ways to protect your health and prevent yourself from potentially deadly health complications like heart attacks. Next join a group or share your concerns with one. You don't have to go it alone.

Action Tips

Weigh yourself every week

Find out or calculate your BMI

Do not stop trying to improve everyday

Do not try to do everything by yourself

Do not try to do everything by yourself. Join a group or form one. This is because no man is an island. It does not have to be a formal group. It could easily be a group made up of family members or friends. Believe me, it is a lot of fun when the whole family is involved in healthy eating and healthy living activities like running and sports events or meets.

Making everybody in your family a part of your healthy living plan is a great idea. If you tell your children that you are no longer going to drink soda with your meals, they will remind you if you forget and try to do it. They will keep you accountable.

Another benefit, you get out of this, is that you start getting into the act of eating healthy. It will be easier to buy milk with reduced fat and get the whole family to eat small carrots and pomegranates.

The next people you need to get into your group will be those in your office whom you share a lunch break with. This way when you think of going for soda, candies and cookies, you will have someone reminding you that you have decided to eat fruits and vegetables during your lunch break. A salad is also a good way to go.

Depending on your budget and personality, you may want to try more formal groups than the ones I have mentioned above. These may be online or offline groups. Whatever group you decide to join, make sure you join a group that suits your personality, your budget and your time.

One major advantage of joining a physical group or becoming part of an online community of people trying to lose weight, is that other people can support you. This can be done by helping you to become more accountable to yourself and others. This can be through reminding you to do your exercise, weigh yourself or even discussing challenges and solutions with a mentor or other group members. Next go over the daily action tips and write down three you will start implementing today. Without action, you will not have results.

Action Tips

Join either a physical group or sign up online to a weight loss membership site or forum

Find out about local running events or sports tournaments in your city and participate in those that interest you

Take action

Join the Compass club @

https://www.facebook.com/compassclub

Daily action tips

UNDERSTAND YOURSELF BETTER

KNOW YOUR PASSION

LEARN YOUR DISC PERSONALITY

KNOW WHAT MOTIVATES YOU

DO A 72-HOUR FOOD AUDIT

CUT DOWN YOUR SERVING PORTIONS

EAT FOOD RICH IN FRUITS AND WHOLE GRAINS

MODIFY YOUR TYPICAL CULTURAL FOOD

DRINK TWO GLASSES OF WATER BEFORE EVERY MEAL

PLAN FOR YOUR SNACKS

CUTDOWN ON SODA AND BEER

READ YOUR NUTRITION FACTS

REDUCE SODIUM INTAKE

REDUCE SUGAR INTAKE

FOCUS ON EATING SLOWLY

**MANAGE YOUR CONVERSATIONS:
YOU DON'T HAVE TO HAVE THE LAST
WORD**

EXERCISE EVERYDAY:

WALK 4 MILES EVERY DAY

SLEEP WELL

TURN OFF YOUR DEVICES

**IMPROVE YOUR EMOTIONAL WELL-
BEING**

IGNORE EMOTIONAL OUTBURSTS

HOPE FOR THE BEST BUT BE PREPARED FOR UNEXPECTED NEGATIVITY DESPITE YOUR BEST INTENTIONS AND ACTIONS

FORGIVE AND FORGIVE AGAIN

FIND AND SAY 10 THANKFUL AND POSITIVE THOUGHTS EVERYDAY

MEASURE YOUR WAIST CIRCUMFERENCE

FIND OUT OR CALCULATE YOUR BMI

A LAPSE IS A NOT A RELAPSE

WEIGH YOURSELF EVERY WEEK

DON'T TRY TO DO EVERYTHING BY YOURSELF

NEVER STOP TRYING TO IMPROVE EVERYDAY

Compass Hybrid Individualized Plan (CHIP)

Here is my own CHIP for weight loss based on the Compass Method for natural weight loss. Remember it does not have to be perfect, you can start with a draft. **My CHIP for weight loss consists of the following 10 steps.**

1, Dedicate at least one hour everyday to exercise through walking, stretching and pushups. Increase my physical activity at work, at home and at leisure. My mini goal is to walk at least 4 miles everyday.

2, Reduce my energy intake everyday by cutting down on my food portion and by increasing my intake of fruits, nuts, and vegetables. Say "No" as many times as possible to processed food and soda.

3, Cut down on daily complaints. I look for other ways to get along instead of focusing on who is wrong or right.

4, Make everyday an opportunity to improve on all aspects of your life. I try to make my daily encounters with people opportunities for learning more about myself and others, so that I can cut down on stress. Why? **When you reduce daily stress, you reduce daily weight gain**.

5, Skip or significantly reduce at least one meal per week.

6, Hold myself accountable by acknowledging my short falls and looking for solutions either by myself or discussing with others. **I weigh myself at least once a week.**

7, Sleep at least 6 hours a day. I do this everyday even if it means breaking it up into smaller periods of time.

8, Avoid comfort snacking or eating to please others. THIS USED TO BE THE BIGGEST REASON WHY I COULD NOT SUSTAIN MY OWN WEIGHT LOSS!!!!

9, Weigh myself everyweek and repeat my food audit at least once a month. Measure my waist circumference every 3 months. **Keep Track!**

10, FOCUS (Follow One Course Until Successful). Follow the Compass Method Until Successful. I remained flexible but never give up on my goal of sustainable weight loss.

There you have it. That is my CHIP for weight loss. Now you can draft yours and share it with us through the Compass Team Facebook group.

Action Tips

Draft your on CHIP for weight loss

Join the Compass club @

https://www.facebook.com/compassclub

Become a member at

http://compasswellnessinstitute.com/membership/

Appendix

BMI=Body mass index. It is a way of assessing your weight and its associated health risks.

DEVELOP YOUR OWN COMPASS HYBRID INDIVIDUALIZED PLAN (CHIP) FOR LOSING WEIGHT AND KEEPING IT OFF

If you have any questions contact me through www.compasswellnessinstitute.com or text 6619926436

What will you do if your diet adjustment strategy fails or you cannot sustain your daily exercise regimen?

Do not give up. Reduce it to what you can do. If you cannot walk 4 miles a day, start with 1 mile a day. Build up slowly. Take care of your mini-goals first.

If you cannot cut down your food portion by half, cut it down by a quarter or by a third.

Add fruits and nuts slowly while you reduce your sodium and sugar intake.

Remember that sustainable change is a slow process. Do not give up on yourself. Don't forget to always consult your doctor and keep your appointments.

Notes

American Heart Association

Anshel, M. H. (2010). The disconnected values
(intervention) model for promoting

healthy

habits in religious institutions. *Journal of*

Religion and Health, 49(1), 32-49. doi:

http://dx.doi.org/10.1007/s10943-008-

9230-x

Bermudez, O. I., Gao, X. (2011, January).
Greater consumption of sweetened
beverages and added sugars is associated
with obesity among US young
adults. *Annals of Nutrition & Metabolism,*
57(3-4) 211-8

CDC2015 Division of nutrition, physical

activity and obesity: Adult obesity facts.

Retrieved from

http://www.cdc.gov/obesity/data/adult.ht
ml

Cleland, V.J., Schmidt , M.D., Dwyer, T., &

Venn, A.J. (2008,May).Television viewing

and abdominal obesity in young adults:

Is the association mediated by food and

beverage consumption during viewing

time or reduced leisure-time physical

activity? *The American Journal of

Clinical Nutrition, 87(5).*

health promotion. *Social Work and*

Christianity, 38(1), 88-100.

Feist, J., & Feist, G. J. (2009). Theories of

Personality (7th ed.). New York:

McGraw-Hill.

Malone, L. (2014).Healthy living: 10 ways your

personality affects your weight. *Huff Post*

online publication

National Heart, Lung and Blood

Institute (NHLBI). (2012).What causes
overweight

and obesity?

Nutrition Research

Reuters Health (2013).Despite obesity rise,

US calories intake trending downwards.

Retrieved from

http://www.reuters.com/article/2013/03/06

/us-despite-obesity-rise-

idUSBRE92518620130306

COMMENTS

PLEASE SHARE YOUR COMMENTS AFTER READING THIS BOOK OR ANY OF MY OTHER BOOKS LISTED IN THE RESOURCES

IF YOU HAVE ANY QUESTIONS OR CONCERNS PLEASE FEEL FREE TO GET IN TOUCH. IF YOU HAVE DEVELOPED YOUR ON CHIP FOR WEIGHT LOSS, PLEASE FILL TO SHARE YOUR SUCCESS STORY WITH US ON FACEBOOK OR ON SEND A TEXT TO ME ON 6619926436.

"Those who succeed are not those who never failed or never missed opportunities but those who never stopped trying."

Dr. Chio Ugochukwu

Resources

Here are additional resources that will help you become the best and happiest version of yourself everyday.

www.compasswellnessinstitute.com

www.compasshealthtransformer.com/members

www.dcompassmarketing.com

http://www.amazon.com/Dr.-Chio-Ugochukwu/e/B00JNFLPQQ

Join the compass club on Facebook

https://www.facebook.com/groups/174827683543 1116/

Other books by Dr. Chio Ugochukwu that will help you improve your health, eliminate stress and transform your life include;

The Compass Health Transformer: Your 72 Hour Blue Print For Healthy Living

21 Ways To Transform Your Health Without Medications

"…21 simple proven ways to reduce stress and improve your health and wellbeing without relying on medications. These are easy and effective ways you can use to turn your daily challenges into transformative opportunities for healthy living and daily happiness. You can start right away without spending a fortune!.."

<u>Get your own copy of 21 Ways To Transform Your Health Without Medications</u>

The Compass Health Transformer Quit Smoking

Overcoming Daily Stress: 21 Quick And Easy Ways To Stay Stress-Free In Your Daily Life

"…Are you tired of being stressed out everyday? Are you tired of feeling exhausted and overwhelmed in your daily activities? Are you fed up with communication issues in your relationship? Here are 21 quick and easy ways you can use to overcome daily stress and turn your daily challenges into opportunities for transformative abundant living. This book will help you gain a better understanding of your potential communication issues, daily 'stress points' and the steps you can take to overcome them…".

Get your own copy of Overcoming Daily Stress

The Secret To Daily happiness

"..Have you ever wondered why daily happiness has continued to elude you? Do you want to make sustainable daily happiness part of your life?

By reading this book. you can find answers to these questions and many more on how to overcome the many obstacles and challenges that daily try to take away your inner peace and contentment..."

Get your own copy of The Secret To Happiness

15 Simple Ways to lower your blood pressure naturally after 40 without complicated diets

"......Don't spend your most productive years dealing with high blood pressure, medications and side effects. Stop worrying about whether you forgot to take your first medication or the second one. Take these simple steps to lower your blood pressure naturally and minimize your need for multiple medications. Did you know that high blood pressure can cause heart attack, stroke, kidney failure, blindness and memory problems? Don't wait to find out! Take Action! ,,,,,"

Click Here for Your own copy of 15 Simple Ways To Reduce Blood Pressure....

Here is a book to help lose fat. If your main concern or focus is losing pounds you have accumulated as fat then get a copy of the book

"How To Lose 23 Pounds of Fat Without Torture Diets or Hard Exercise And keep it (The Compass Method).

"Are you fed up with trying to lose weight again and again with limited success? Are you tired of all the confusing new and expensive diets you have tried to follow every day with zero results? Do you want the health benefits of living with optimum weight without following complicated rules? Do you want to become more energtic and active again? Are you fed up with the wild ride of losing weight today and gaining it back tomorrow? Then read this book so that you will start using a comprehensive individualized weight loss strategy that will help you lose fat and keep it off, without going on torture diets or deadly strenuous exercises. You will learn to do this through the Compass Method that is based on a holistic approach to weight-loss, healthy living and personal transformation."

If prayer is something that appeals to you, you might be interested in the following next two books that incorporate prayers into our daily strive to become better and become more fulfilled:

Praying To Win: How To Get More Victories And Riches In Your Daily Life Through Spiritual Principles

"..You too can achieve your goals and dreams, through praying to win. You can do this by immersing yourself in the word of God and transforming the moments that make up your daily life through persistent adoration……. Above all, thank God everyday, never give up and persistently continue praying to win..."

Get your own copy of Praying To Win

9 Best Ways To Eliminate Stress, Improve Your Health And thrive Without Limitations Through Prayers

Are tired of being knocked down by stress from your daily hassles? Are you tired of dealing with chronic illnesses associated with stress? Do you want to live a fun-filled daily life? Here are 9 of the best ways you can change your daily obstacles and challenges into opportunities to thrive without limitations through the power of prayers.

Too Young To Die

"A book about coping with grief and finding your way in life…"

9 Best Ways To Quit Smoking Without Becoming A Nervous Wreck And Gaining Weight

"..Here are 9 of the best ways to finally quit smoking without becoming a nervous wreck or gaining weight. If you have tried to quit smoking before, but failed or tried to quit but was overcome by anxiety or fear of becoming socially awkward or gaining weight, then read this book! This book was previously published as "The Compass Health Transformer Quit Smoking", but has been rewritten to include the transtheoretical model of change to help you get a better understanding of where you are in your journey or process of quitting smoking. The 9 best ways to quit smoking also includes a reminder of the different ways smoking can affect your health and body and the different individualized-changes you can make to your life-style to help you quit smoking on your own terms.

9 Best Ways To Deal With Negative People, Protect Your Health And Be Happy

"..Are you tired of being stressed out by encounters with negative people? Are you fed up with the impact of negative situations on your health and happiness? Would like you to find out ways to remain effective during negative situations and encounters with negative people? Do you know that chronic stress generated by negative encounters can damage your eyes, heart and brain? Do you know that chronic stress can directly damage your body cells? Here are 9 best ways you can protect your health from such negative situations so that you can continue to thrive and be happy..".

To order new or additional copies or ask questions, please visit:

http://www.amazon.com/Dr.-Chio-Ugochukwu/e/B00JNFLPQQ

Call or Text : 661 992 6436

You can also get EBOOKS from

www.compasswellnessinstitute.com/Ebooks

Join the Compass club @

https://www.facebook.com/compassclub

Here is the back cover quote:

"Your present circumstances don't determine where you can go; they merely determine where you start."

Nido Qubein

About the Author

Dr. Chio Ugochukwu has always been interested in helping people improve their health, eliminate stress, transform their lives, and become the best and happiest versions of themselves. He has dedicated his life to helping individuals and organizations use data to improve their health outcomes through more effective intrapersonal and interpersonal communications. He has always been interested in helping others improve themselves, become more empowered in their search for better health, more success and greater happiness despite their busy schedules, daily activities and duties.

He was inspired to develop the Compass Method, through the challenges he has encountered in his journey of life, his practice of medicine and his fascination with how effective communications, the mind, the spirit and human experience influence the fulfillment of life. You can find out more about the Compass Method and other membership groups by Dr Chio by visiting www.compasswellnessinstitute.com.

As an author and researcher, he has published many books, with peer-reviewed publications on quality of life and numerous articles on transformational living. He is the medical director of Dala Compass Foundation and a consultant with the Compass Consultants International (CCI). As a consultant and health communications strategist, he is focused on sharing with individuals and organizations, customized methods and strategic pathways for improving health and getting the best performance for themselves and their organizations.

www.ingramcontent.com/pod-product-compliance
Lightning Source LLC
Chambersburg PA
CBHW071201280526
45787CB00002B/564